Take a Deep Breath

Diary of a Junior Doctor in the NHS

During the Covid Pandemic

By

Dr. Talha Sami
MBBS iBSc MA MRCGP

Take a Deep Breath

www.drtsami.com
Portfolio

www.sofarunsaid.com
SFU focusses on delivering an alternative narrative for those less-explored stories through podcasts, documentaries and interviews

www.iconsultplus.com
See our highly experienced specialist psychiatrists, psychologists or our general medical consultant at your own comfort

www.passtherca.com
The most comprehensive resources needed to pass the Remote Consultation Assessment for MRCGP

Take a Deep Breath offers a refreshingly honest account of what it's like to be an aspiring doctor whose professional life and marriage get turned upside down by the pandemic.

Dr. Jeremy Howick
Director of the Oxford University Empathy Programme and author of Doctor You

I met Talha during his GP training scheme in Guildford; due to the Coronavirus pandemic the final six months of his training were not as anyone expected - not only did all teaching initially get cancelled but was later reinstated in a virtual format. Talha found himself one of the first cohort sitting the new RCGP RCA examination. This was challenging to say the least.

Dr. Debra Harper
GP Partner and GP Training Programme Director

This was a time of great unrest and uncertainty but in the space of a few weeks Talha prepared for and successfully sat the new RCA. He learnt much over this time and was extremely quick to condense his learning to support fellow registrars keen to know more about this exam. As his trainer I am delighted by Talha's energy and motivation.

Dr. Charlotte Knight
GP Partner and GP Trainer

Take a Deep Breath

Do men think that they will be left alone because they say, 'we believe' and that they will not be tested?

The Holy Quran
Chapter 23: The Spider

Acknowledgements

The list of individuals to whom I am grateful spans many years and institutions. I am humbled and truly privileged to have had these remarkable figures in my life.

I have cherished Dr. Christina Baboonian's incredible support for almost fifteen years which started as my tutor whilst I was at St. George's, University of London when I was studying medicine. I am indebted to Dr. Jeremy Howick for the time we spent at UCL: he helped mould my critical reasoning skills and intellect. Alas I would not be where I am without what I learnt then. Whilst studying for my Master's at SOAS Dr. Jan-Peter Hartung pushed me further than I ever thought I could go.

Dr. Charlotte Knight has been incredibly supportive for as long as I have known her; more than I could ever have asked for. Dr. Debra Harper and Dr. Fiona Groom warrant notable mention for the times they put up with me and the advice they gave over the past few years. Dr. Martin Brunet guided me through the writing process. I should acknowledge Dr. Arrigo, Dr. Marican and Mr Schneider who have cultivated my passion for Emergency Medicine. I am thankful for Dr. Ozan Hanci for the time, support and tutelage he has provided me.

Out of all my friends (who all play their own very important roles in my life) I would like to single out Kareem who has been a superlative role model, tremendous friend and fantastic inspiration for many years. He has enthused me with a passion for my studies, politics, humanitarian efforts and helped me realise the importance of my day-to-day work. Finally I must of course mention my loving, nurturing family who have supported me and guided me all my life.

Author's Introduction

This is an inside look into the front-line response of the pandemic recorded in real-time. It chronicles my failures, stresses, romance, frailty, mental health, life and death in the worst health crisis of the past hundred years. 2020 was a monumental year for so many people in so many ways. There were so many things that caught our attention – these included the American presidential elections, the death of George Floyd and of course the worldwide coronavirus pandemic.

It appears the NHS has always been under stress and tension. This was put into hyperdrive by the coronavirus pandemic which rapidly snowballed into something unprecedented. Every day key workers show up is a monumental tribute to how strong these workers are and the healthcare system. I believe it's the best healthcare system in the world. I passionately feel it's what makes my country the best country in the world despites the shortcomings.

This was the year that held so many highs and lows for me. I was getting married, ready to move in with my bride, gain some seniority in my A&E role and become a GP. This was all derailed in some way or another. I failed my last exam I needed to pass to become a GP. The marriage was postponed – it was delayed several times because of the ongoing pandemic. I saw Pernia infrequently during the first wave. It took a toll on me mentally. I had to look within to become stronger to combat the external ever-changing environment. I had dreams of starting a business and writing a passion project on the religious history in America. All of this fell to the wayside.

This book opens up with my nervous anticipation of getting ready to sit my final exam to become a GP. I observed coronavirus from a distance; it ravaged European health systems before it came to England. We worked through the uncertainties of trying to manage a disease we didn't know and frankly had little idea about; I was trying to balance my own personal affairs of my career progression and marriage at the same time. It took a toll on my mental health; I felt the effects and my anxiety building. I had all the nervousness and worries any groom-to-be would have. I had concerns about living with a vulnerable mother who previously had cancer. I had my own health concerns too.

Having been brought up around a psychiatrist mother and brother I have a passion for re-thinking mental health. These journals were meant to be private. It was a cathartic release to retain my sanity. I wanted to keep them in their original form as much as possible. What you read is a lived experience which comes alive in script: it was crucial to keep any raw emotion no matter how visceral. If there is an odd phrase, atypical sentence or even incorrect grammar that is a reflection of how I felt then. The awkward statements and imprecise syntax poured forth. In hindsight I think there are many things that would benefit the reader. I believe that healthcare workers have become marginalised and dehumanised; people forget that we're not superheroes and not just dogsbodies. We are frequently stressed in a highly pressured environment. We have our own personal responsibilities; often our domestic lives can be in array because of what goes on. Our health suffers and our relationships too. I think these diaries begin to show that.I would like to think this is a tale of perseverance but I'll leave that to you to decide. Eventually I did pass my exam and become a GP. I was promoted in the Emergency Department at a time when the country needed it so much. I did finally get married. My wife began her own work as a junior doctor and Pernia writes her own stories in the follow-up to this entitled *I Need A Second Opinion* which chronicles our journey through the second wave of the pandemic together.

I'm writing this introduction at the time of the second wave. We are in the eye of the storm. I'm tired; I feel my resilience eroding. The vaccine gives me hope and my colleagues give me hope; looking at the NHS makes me proud but at the same time I survey the damage that 30 to 40 years of privatisation and systematic de-funding has done.

I believe this is a story that strongly needs to be told. It needs to be heard by as many people as possible. I think the last year has shown that we are all closer together than we think we are.

Dr. Talha Sami
MBBS iBSc MA MRCGP
1st January 2021

2nd January 2020

My first diary entry of the year. Where do I start? It looks like a great year ahead. I'm hopefully finishing my exams and becoming a GP soon. It's booked for February; if I pass it the rest of the year should be smooth sailing.

I look forward to moving in with Pernia. 31 December 2018 was when I first met her – it was at her home. I had just got back from America a few days before and it was scheduled relatively quickly. I was then flying to Pakistan in a few days to volunteer in a hospital. It seems so long ago now. I met her family and her too. She seemed very sweet and innocent; she was friendly and respectable – that's what she said about me in fact when I first met her! Her family and her brothers seemed really nice too.

She is currently finishing her final medical year. I really liked that she was educated, friendly and polite. I specifically remember we talked about our faith; she said her prayers were very important for her. For me that was really important.

I then met her next a few weeks later. I think within a few months I knew she was the one who I wanted to marry. Traditionally Muslims don't date but we do get to know one another and the family on an intimate basis. We frankly discussed future lifestyles and plans. We seemed to get on. Really feel very fortunate that I met her. I feel very blessed and am excited about spending my life with her.

She was the one I had been waiting for a long time. We often talk about "the one". It seems like a mythical concept at times. When I discovered in Islam that there is that perfect partner, I was pleasantly surprised. The only way that partner can be found is through prayer and not through our own human efforts which are often flawed and wrought with human emotion. 100% I stand by that. I've been very fortunate and blessed.

We've got our wedding scheduled in the summer. I know she is very excited; as is my mum too. Weddings always seem to be a lady's affair!

I just see potential. I look forward to having my own life back and not working on the rota anymore. I look forward to being my own boss. I look forward to spending time with my wife. I have so many goals I want to achieve. I'm working on a three-volume series on religion in America over the past century, which I have been doing for the past couple of years now. Research is slow but I'm trying to push through every day doing it bit by bit.

My focus is trying to pass this next exam. I want to work on my diet and try and increase my faith I'm always trying to self-evaluate and re-evaluate to make sure I've given my best.

Definitely I've got a lot of weaknesses; I'm far too ambitious. I don't always take into account my limitations. Most definitely I have felt that at times too.

18th January 2020

I am a little bit anxious about this exam but it will be over soon. We get told that it's the final exam we will ever do as GPs. No more exams ever! It's 13 different practical scenarios; I have been revising since October of last year with two of my peers. I think we're all prepared to be honest. I really have tried to put in the work. However even at medical school I would always work consistently; I would never cram because that would never benefit me. That was completely different to the other students.

I've been revising with friends. I attended a course. I've worked hard on trying to really touch up my communication skills and take on all the attributes my superiors have told me about. It's definitely a lot of effort. I've been revising for about 3-4 months whilst most people started later; most people won't sit the exam as early as February given that our year starts in August.

I've had some back pain recently. I think it's to do with the long drives to when I go to see Pernia. To be honest it's really nice to go to West London; I don't go that often. I enjoy the drive and I enjoy spending time with her family too. I've spent so much time in South London studying and living there. It's nice to learn about West London – it has so much rich history and flavour. Love it.

It's really annoying though that my back pain is constantly there. If I'm honest I've never really experienced anything like this before; it does make me empathise a little bit more with people who suffer with continual back pain. I don't want to take tablets – I didn't really understand when people said that before but now I do. I think this might be a result of not working out my legs at the gym! I think partially it's also growing older and the working life taking a toll. It's just so different being on the other side and needing help. I had to go through the whole process of going to the GP and being referred.

It's a lot better with physiotherapy. I'm just so glad I had a quick referral and the physiotherapist was so helpful. I think that's so wonderful in the NHS. I do get some issues with my back from time to time. I think this merely made me appreciate the services that we have. I have another appointment booked as well. I didn't really understand the logic behind the physiotherapy; they taught me leg exercises when I had lower back pain but now I can see the sense of it. It really made a difference.

Also, on the same note my heartburn is a little bit better. I tried to change my diet a little bit too. I just think I feel the effects of age. I definitely drink too much coffee and I do overeat. I'm not the only person that's made this observation about myself. I'm trying to watch that – it's quite difficult in a GP lifestyle when there are always lots of treats in the kitchen.

Self-discipline is key.

22nd January 2020

I need to just be calm at all times. That's kind of one thing that I've seen – you can't always perform at the highest level all the time. Even a top athlete steps in and out of that zone. It is about being mentally sharp at all times.

That's where rest comes in.

I recently started buying some perfumes and colognes. Trying to move up the style ladder; be a little more stylish. I've made it a little thing. I really find it is a nice release and it's wonderful to stimulate the senses and treat yourself from time to time.

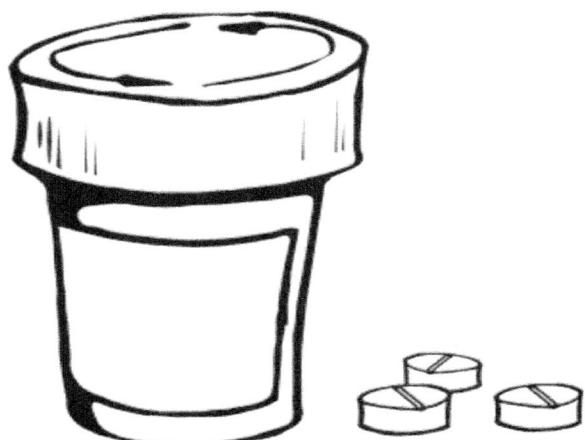

I'm thinking about what to do after this exam. Probably add some more Emergency Medicine shifts and develop my skills. I definitely want to work on my faith. I would like to try and go jogging and develop my GP skills too. Seems all is falling into place. I'm trying to read more and fast more as well.

One of my dreams is to work as a doctor abroad. I've done that a few times already – I worked in Pakistan, West Africa and Calais in austere environments. These were experiences in themselves. I want to be a master – I want to be the best A&E doctor and the best GP. That way I can treat everything.

I've been fortunate I've been able to travel so much. I travelled the world twice in 2015 and 2018; 2015 I worked in the camps in Calais. I'll be honest I felt way out of my depth. The nurses there did far better than me and were much more comfortable. We had limited supplies. I went to The Gambia twice in 2015 and 2016 with Humanity First – I would like to think our medical team made a difference there. We renovated one of the A&E rooms and stocked it full. The next time we went back the doctors said they were using it as a major trauma room. It had worked. The paediatric team especially had made a difference. I wish I could go back but it's been tricky to get the time off to go.

Sometimes when you're in the grind, you know everything seems a bit monotonous. You just have to keep going. There are little victories here and there. It's nice to think about the future. I don't think my future has ever looked so bright so I'm very thankful for that.

6th February 2020

Something happened recently where a patient complained about the treatment that I had given them; they were not happy. The incident was a year ago but this was only raised now. I had to write a short report and de-brief with my consultant. I was quite taken aback by this – so were my colleagues who I informed about this.

I guess I learnt my lesson. Always be clear with patients; sometimes we take too much of a doctor-centric approach and that does not always work.

I ran this by some of my colleagues too. They didn't really understand the nature of the complaint either. It's really devastating when a patient complains; I generally think that as doctors we were mostly higher achievers at school (that does not apply to me though. I feel I was middle of the road in so many ways) so when something goes wrong then that can be quite heart-breaking. Whenever I've made a mistake, I dwell on it a lot. I don't let it settle. It makes my stomach turn over.

At the same time, I need to learn. I take criticism really badly; I'm working on trying to improve. Maybe that's common for everyone?

I think people don't really see us as people all the time; we are really stretched with resources as it already is. I understand though because they're in pain and upset so they want someone to hear them out. It goes both ways. *"Patients want to be heard"* my trainer tells me. Very true.

I've been doing a lot of calculation recently about trying to figure out how the honeymoon and all my other expenses would work. Obviously, there is a marriage coming soon too. Having to save up a little bit of money before Pernia moves in too.

We were thinking about different locations to go. My dentist mentioned she went to Santorini recently, Greece; the pictures look phenomenal! I know one of my friends went to the Amalfi Coast in Italy too. That's in the mix as well.

Trying to figure it out is quite a big task. Enjoyable though.

I didn't realise getting married was so expensive!

12th February 2020

I am nervous about the exam. I don't want to live in that space though. I want to execute at the highest level possible. At all times. Easier said than done.

I've been revising with some of my colleagues recently. Sometimes I feel okay but sometimes I feel nervous. I did some revision with an old friend of mine who recently did the exam – he really shook me up. I remember we were eating out and I thought I would try run my game face by him and my approach. I couldn't even eat my food properly after we were done and my stomach was in knots.

People have so much different information and different views about this exam that it makes it really hard to know how to go forward. Practical exams are always a little unpredictable and everyone has a different experience so there's nothing linear about it.

I can't underestimate how important this exam is. That being said I'm definitely taking it way too seriously. Some people say we all seem to overhype it. I think as medical students studying was a very big thing and it was a competitive environment. That never really left us. Frankly though, I do not think there is always a correlation between doing well at medical school and being a good doctor – it goes a lot deeper than book knowledge. Implementation of knowledge and communication skills are equally as important. These are things we learn with experience sometimes.

All I know is that I've done my best thus far. Exam's only a few days away now. The waiting is the worst. Just want it to be over and done with now.

13th February 2020 (pre-exam)

Last night I got to Central London quite late. The exam is this morning; I'm staying near the exam centre so I'm fresh.

Back in my old area; I'm really familiar with this area. I went to UCL for a year and I studied at SOAS. I remember walking down to Covent Garden and chilling out there a number of times. I did my Philosophy degree at UCL during my medical degree. That was when mum was ill; I didn't really get much out of the university experience and it was quite a trek to get to Central for my classes. I really didn't pay much attention to my studies that year. My brother was very helpful with my dissertation then.

Years later when I was at SOAS, I really enjoyed my time there. It was an amazing experience and one that I will never forget. I met so many friends and learnt so much. I loved all the experiences, and it was incredible studying in such an academic institution in Central London. Being here is bringing back memories. One of the best experiences of my life – that being said I remember working on weekends, studying in the evenings and socialising. It cost a lot of money and time. Living on the knife-edge in some ways. I loved it though.

It's funny that my mum went to Birkbeck as well decades before. Treading the same paths…

I really didn't sleep overnight. The bed was really quite hard. There was a little bit of noise, as to be expected. In fact, I didn't sleep at all I don't think. I had a thorough breakfast. I just want to get this over and done with.

Journaling really keeps me level. Takes the nerves away.

It's exam day. I do think I've got some composure. I'm not living in a negative space. I think I'm downplaying my tensions.

It'll be over in a few hours and there's so much to look forward to as well.

13th February 2020 (post-exam)

Done!

I've done my best. I worked as hard as I could. I prayed about it as well. Overall, I think I definitely made mistakes but I think it was only in three parts of it. I think I've done enough to pass.

Who doesn't run out of time on their exams? I think it was a fair exam. I was able to do the relevant data gathering and communicate my concerns alongside my treatment appropriately. I think the patients felt heard.

I'm very fortunate with my trainer and teacher; she has had decades of experience. I do think as well I tried to take on a lot of her softer skills that I did not have before. I think my knowledge was there and is strong but I do think my communication skills are a little bit too hard at times. I think I did what I needed to do.

This year I learnt a lot about being a GP; the main thing is learning to communicate. Who would think we have to learn that? That's the biggest key skill. It's also helped temper my own emotions and made me a better human. Being aware of our emotions and how we express them I mean; so often I can get it wrong. Mindfulness is really beneficial although I don't practise it enough.

I was revising with a colleague online who sat the exam too; as soon as we came out, he said I think *"I've fluffed it"*. I felt confident. I felt like I should console him. Maybe he was being over-anxious. I was surprised that he felt that way. When we talked about what we encountered he had different information to me when comparing answers – that worried me.

14th February 2020

I'm just waiting for results now. Honestly, I think I passed.

What more can I have done? I just want to be prepared and never take anything for granted. I do think it was a fair exam.

I keep re-evaluating every exam scenario. I did it on the train/tube on the way back home. Then I went through it all with my trainer as well at a later date. She said it sounds like you did what you needed to do but she did mention some concerns over two or three things that I may have missed. She didn't give me 100% assurance. I guess that she can't of course.

Just sit and wait.

21st February 2020

Recently I was a bit worried that I missed something or something was not done right in regards to patient care. These are the kinds of things that we take home with ourselves. Then we constantly keep thinking about these things. Often it takes a lot more work to be safe and we end up staying late but that's the sacrifice we have to make.

This is the thing. I'm still learning. I'm always still learning. I have a long way to go. I definitely am not the finished product but I know that I'm almost there. There are things here and there that I will miss.

Someone once said to me that *"you don't want to go home and worry about someone"*. I've often noticed if I stay half an hour or an hour later and tie up all the loose ends then I go home comfortable. I think that's just our call of duty; we obviously don't get paid for overtime but what we are doing is very noble, as my mum keeps reminding me. I guess she is saying that from her own experience of being a consultant for over 20 years.

I have to just keep going. I'm thinking about the marriage ceremony and work at the minute. Lots to look forward to.

Keep going…
Results coming soon…

23rd February 2020

I failed.

I found out a short while ago. I had just come out of the mosque and sat in my car after evening prayers. Anxiously I was checking the results on my phone and kept re-loading the screen. I remember feeling confident…

I checked my phone and I then double-checked the results. I texted Pernia immediately – she was quite reassuring. She was telling me about my father-in-law who failed his exams a number of times when he was becoming a surgeon. He had an incredibly tough time. He's the sweetest too.

I was going to meet my friends after passing – I will have to cancel that. I had some business plans; I will have to cancel that. I was planning on doing a few more courses about general practice. I'm going to have to cancel that too. I had some ideas about work and doing some more shifts; I'll have to cancel that too.

I'm going to have to sit down and commit myself to revision. Might have to sit down and think when do I want to sit this exam?

This is really tough given that two of my colleagues passed. I was revising with them and felt I was on their level too. Obviously, I'm upset but I need to think of the positives; I look forward to getting married. I look forward to just having a job, having my physical and mental health when so many people don't.

I always want to turn my losses into victories. How can I do that? I will do a breakdown of all of my physical, financial, medical habits and work on each area.

There needs to be some meaning to all of this. I need to find a reason why I failed. Otherwise, it's just pointless – not getting anything from it. I have to learn a lesson. It's just easier said than done and I really can't see the logic behind all of this either.

I remember once my mum said to me when her cousin died *"where was the logic in that?"* It was just something we had to accept. That's when we're tested.

Sometimes things are just a test and we are tested.

We have to come out on the other side.

Really quite heart-broken…

25th February 2020

Here's a breakdown:
I have split my life into physical training, spirituality and finances. I need to work on each of those aspects to develop something further. I need a new me. I need a new focus.

I take failure and criticism really hard. I don't take them well. I need to work on that. One of my many weaknesses.

On the flipside it's just an exam; it's really hard to hear that because my whole life focussed around passing this exam. I just feel so fortunate that everything else has gone okay, I guess.

I think about how my mum was ill.
I think about when I was trying to get into medical school.
I think about all the difficulties that I had.
I think about when I didn't have money before starting work.

I'm grateful that so many other things have sorted themselves out. I'm sure this will too. It's hard to see that far ahead in the future. Sometimes it's hard to keep going and it's hard to keep the faith.

Sometimes it's hard to persevere.

25th February 2020

How do I make a negative positive?

How do I make failure a success?

How do I close the gap?

How do I adapt to failure?

Question after question swirling around my mind.

27th February 2020

I'm really trying to overhaul my lifestyle by fasting regularly. Increasing the amount of time at the gym. I'm working towards finishing my exams and becoming a GP. Hopefully by August 2020.

Recently I was thinking a bit deeper. I remember I saw a disabled person that was wheeled into the canteen. I remember looking at them while that person tried to eat but their hands were too short or they couldn't manoeuvre to put the food in their mouth. We take things like our mobility for granted. So much. I just saw this for a split second; however, they have to live like that and live in that wheelchair. I'm sure that person lives a happy life (I hope they do) but I'm sure they have it tough from time to time. We should all be more grateful.

Recently I found out something very sad – there was a boy who I went to school with who was a few years above me. He went to my medical school also. He was a really nice guy and I remember when I bumped into him from time to time, he would give me advice. I saw him as a junior doctor when I was still a student; at that point he gave me advice. He offered good tips and even offered to help me too. That was the last time I saw him. It was many years ago now.

Someone else mentioned him to me too in the past year. We talked about how this individual had suffered with a Crohn's disease. I did not know that. Often it's controllable; however, he had to have multiple operations for it. He had an extremely severe, unrelenting form of this disease. I imagine it must have affected him mentally throughout his years as a junior doctor. I'd also found out he was now working in London as a GP trainee a few years ago; so he was above me by a few years.

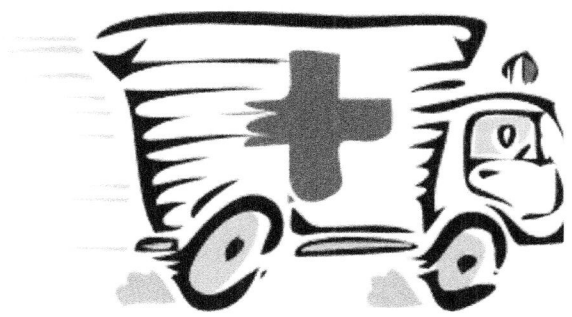

Then I went on a course where someone mentioned a doctor working in East London had tragically died. For some reason I searched his name. It was a sad and shocking moment.

I never heard one person say anything bad about him throughout our various interactions of school, medical school and at work. He had multiple operations since the age of seven. In his final year of becoming a GP he could not eat any more from what I gathered. He had to have nutrition fed into his veins. He would regularly have to go to empty his stoma bag multiple times during his A&E shifts.

Later I gathered that he died of a cardiac arrest caused by sepsis at the age of 31. He had just got married… How am I different right now? That could have been me.

Makes me feel overwhelmed with gratitude about what I have. This is very sad about this young man and his family.

I get so caught up in the little things in the day today and I don't really think about the big things and the bigger picture.

Rest in peace, old friend…

29th February 2020

I'm still in development.
I'm still trying to add in changes and make them a part of my life.
Adding new habits takes time and I'm definitely going to make mistakes on the way.

I really like the 80/20 rule. You love yourself 80% of the time.
The other 20% you have to be tough on yourself.

Anything more than that makes it too difficult either way.

1st March 2020

The Arabic word for disaster (مصيبة) often indicates catastrophe but there is timing and perfection embedded in the etymological part of it. What we get is what is meant to happen. It's the mentality which is where I need to change.

We can only control ourselves and not the environment.

Once I said these kinds of things to my cousin and he said it sounds like more like you're saying it to yourself than it factually being true. I don't think that's true. It is reassuring to me to think like this when I review things.

I'm a scientist and I believe in empirical data; I react to facts and data. At the same time the human mind is irrational and emotional. Life is very much about constraining / restraining our desires and fears.

The way I'm looking at it right now is that May will be Ramadan. June will be the wedding and the honeymoon.

What wonderful times.

2nd March 2020

I'm trying to work on my jogging and physical training. Have advanced a lot in the last few days. I dread jogging though!

My goal is always to go to bed satisfied knowing I've done absolutely everything I need to do that day.

It's nice to see all these positive entries after failing the exam. I just want to push forward. Makes failing a reason that something has happened. I can pinpoint that as the change. That's what made me be better.

4th March 2020

I'm looking forward to June when the wedding is. We already had the Islamic rituals and rites of passage. There are a few more cultural celebrations the family would like to do. It's nice to see my mum occupied with this.

Sometimes it's easier to go with the flow.

When you fight against tension it doesn't actually ease the tension. What I mean is when there is tension and you pull it, it creates more tension. If you ease up lightly then that eases the tension. It never seems to benefit meeting stress with more stress.

That's one thing that I really admire about Emergency Medicine doctors; in particular the consultants. I have never once seen them stressed. Never worn down. They're constantly calm and able to deal with information in abundance. No matter where I worked or with whom.

My dream goal is to get a promotion in this line of work from a junior level in the emergency department to a more senior level. That would mean becoming a registrar; I don't think I'm too far off that at the minute, as I have the right qualifications. I believe I've got the experience I need but maybe I need more. I look forward to trying to work on this.

7th March 2020

I'm literally counting the days down to the exam. I've booked it again to re-sit it.

I gave myself enough space which is about two months from failing originally. I think that's enough time for me to work on whatever weaknesses I have. I am still a little bit baffled by the whole procedure but I can only carry on. I was thinking of some of my friends from medical school who are far brighter than me; they actually failed the same exam as well. That was a real surprise to me.

I'm not really sure how much more I can change. I went through everything with my trainer and other doctors too. I can only do my best. I have re-booked it and I'll see what happens.

I find the stress eases by enjoying my leisure time – this has included watching some TV and catching up with friends. I think originally, I had a proper knee-jerk reaction which was to cancel everything. That's not healthy.

8th March 2020

Was nice to catch up with old friends; I get so caught up in my own mind. I often live in my own head. It's really lovely to spend time with old friends to see where we were and where we are now.

One thing I have noticed is that I need to work on my diet! I often see doctors, including myself, have a really tough time controlling their diets. I think it's to do with long hours. It's tough to stay in shape particularly with ageing metabolism. I need to commit myself to a better diet and new physical training. Just need that mental strength needed to keep a consistently clean diet whilst not giving into snacking.

Maybe that's the nature of all competitive and high-powered jobs. You have to sacrifice parts of yourself and give that to the job. I'm near the end of the tunnel where I can control my life and everything much more. Hopefully I can manoeuvre things to my favour.

I think the dream for everyone is to be in charge of their timetable. I see that more and more with the millennial generation where they want to work part-time. I want to work from home to be more in control of things. It's very different to what I remember my parents going through where they were committed and they were thoroughbreds in their fields. It was all encompassing for them. I think the same is the case with my grandfather too and that was thousands of miles away in Pakistan almost a century ago.

10th March 2020

I feel happier.

I've got five months to go until my freedom.

Three months until I move in with Pernia.

11th March 2020

"He would leave nothing in the tank"

Someone said that about Kobe. What an attitude and what a way to live. I still think about how incredible an athlete he was, even though it's been 2 months since his death.

I do feel anxious about the exam coming. It's put me into an introspective mood. I reflect back and remember when I was in my twenties. I was making a lot of mistakes. Much of this was to do with impulsivity. I just didn't want to listen to other people and I thought I knew best. Does that sound familiar?

I need to try and make negatives positives. I was felt there was a guiding hand to take me away from that. That same force pointed me towards the positive. I think the twenties are a time when we make a lot of mistakes. Once when I was on my paediatric rotation, my supervisor said to me *"people change a lot in their twenties"*. How true. I just look back at myself with stark apathy and contempt because I was really headed in the wrong direction. I feel really blessed just to be where I am now.

Course I'm worried about failing in my exam again – then extending my training and disrupting my plans. It's interesting that we plan so many things but then what happens? We have to react to life. Our plans don't always pan out.

It's becoming official. The World Health Organisation declared the coronavirus a pandemic today. I think this is going to start having a massive impact now like never before. Let's see what happens.

Every moment is another opportunity to review what I'm doing wrong and what I'm doing right.

12th March 2020

I'm looking forward to this exam being over. I kept a fast today for health and spiritual reasons. I'm trying to do this fasting once a week. There are so many benefits to it. It's like a detox for me.

Looking forward to all the wedding functions in three months and then having my freedom in five months!

Sometimes I don't have a lot to report!

14th March 2020

The first death from coronavirus was confirmed on the 5th March. I think the number of cases has exceeded 100.

Then by 7th March the cases went over 200. It was on the 12th of March when the UK Chief Medical Officers raised the risk from moderate to high – the government advised anyone with a new, continuous cough or fever should isolate for seven days. There are major changes afoot. This is all happening very quickly in terms of the governmental changes.

Recently one of my friends asked me what I make of this coronavirus thing when we were driving through Clapham. Mirra took me to a new burger place; I think it was last month. I said I think it's just a hype and there was no need to be worried. It's gotten a lot more serious since then and I've eaten my words. This thing seems to be rapidly taking over the whole world and affecting all life.

Although it came out of nowhere – I don't think anyone anticipated this. I mean even with the warning signs; it seems that it's ramped up very quickly.

We've been warned that the exam will be cancelled most likely. It's quite likely the wedding may not go ahead; I know my mum put her heart and soul into this. She spent a lot of money trying to organise this. Same with Pernia; she was really excited about it. I literally have nowhere else to turn to. This is where faith comes in…

15th March 2020

I've got a little bit of tension about the exam. I've booked it. It is the final exam I will have to do. It's not clear what's going to happen right now though.

Similarly, what does this all mean for the wedding? I mean will it get cancelled? What will happen to my training this year? If I passed the exam and I got through the rest of the year then I could be a GP by August. It's unclear exactly what's going to happen.

Also, Ramadan is coming soon. I'm trying to plan out a diet to keep myself going in. This is a tough time. Plus, these will be long days to be fasting in.

16th March 2020

I got an email today that the exam is cancelled. I guess I'm happy that I know now. It was unclear what was going to happen because some individuals sat the exam this Saturday, right before it was cancelled.

It's likely the wedding has been delayed and the holiday will be cancelled. We will have to wait to see how it plays out and what will happen. I mean will we have to push the functions back a lot? Will we have to have a smaller function? I don't know.

All of this is spiralling out of control. Mentally I'm going to have to try and shift my focus and my landscape; these are clearly things out of my control now and I need to accept what comes.

Stay strong.
Stay flexible.

17th March 2020

I'm worried about what happens with our exam, the honeymoon and the marriage.

Of course, Pernia is really quite upset about everything being thrown off. She only visited Pakistan recently over the winter to get all her dresses made. It's an unwritten rule that all Pakistani girls have to go to Pakistan to get their wedding clothes made to bring them back. Now it looks like none of this may even happen.

She spent a month there which is the longest time for her; she hasn't been back in a very long time and even then, she was quite busy daily. She wasn't even able to respond to me regularly when she got there!

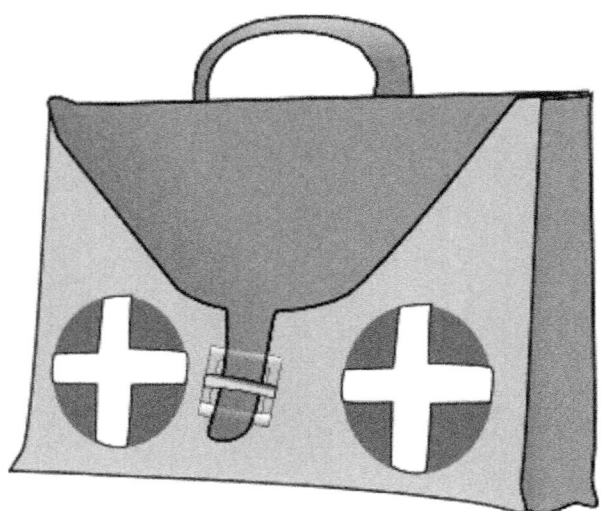

19th March 2020

It's difficult to predict how long all of this is going to last for. I'm imagining a couple of months. Maybe I'm being foolishly optimistic here. I guess we never really have dealt with anything of this size.

At the same time I believe strongly in fate. Everything is written and everything is perfectly weighted. Whatever the challenges; we need to be prepared for them.

We need to be mentally in the right frame to deal with them. I get so caught up in planning every day, week, month and year but ultimately so many things happen that are out of control. The most successful people are those that can adapt to different circumstances and environments. Ultimately that's what success is. It's foolish to think that we can control everything. In fact, this often leads to a crippling realisation when things don't go right.

It's easier to be loose and manoeuvrable.

22nd March 2020

Coronavirus!

There is definitely a lot of uncertainty now in regard to many things. I think our governing bodies will figure out what to do for an exam. There is definitely a delay to the wedding. It looks like a honeymoon is going to get cancelled. I'm waiting to see where Pernia gets her job.

Our family gathered together to watch the PM's announcement. There's almost an awe of suspended disbelief.

Our practice was mostly doing telephone triage anyway. I am having to come in an extra day a week. That makes things a little tougher.

Surprisingly work has been really quiet so far. We don't really have that many requests to see anyone. I guess we are dealing with the first wave and we will have to see how that changes.

By 20th March I think the worldwide death toll had surpassed 10,000. I don't think we really have felt the full effects yet. This seems to be progressing very rapidly. Are we prepared enough?

Keep going as you are.

26th March 2020

Lockdown. The roads are quiet. The shops are shut.

All of our family sits down regularly together to watch Boris talk about the lockdown. This is the first time we've spent together in some time. We're looking at the briefings whenever they occur.

What's going to happen to the wedding? What's going to happen to the honeymoon? What's going to happen to my training?

Lots of uncertainty. I think globally cases have reached 500,000 by today. This is becoming like a snowball effect; things just seem to be worsening quickly.

I had a chat with my trainer recently; she said even in her decades of her experience she's never seen anything like this. We are truly in uncharted waters.

A new scheme started called 'Clap For Carers'. I think it's wonderful, it's so heart-warming to know the average public comes out to support us. It makes a real difference knowing that we are appreciated. People are coming out, even banging pots and pans, just to say thank you. How wonderful!

1st April 2020

I think a lot of the tensions right now arise due to the uncertainty.

I don't know what's going to happen with the honeymoon or the holiday. I was quite looking forward to going to Santorini. I'm obviously looking at the travel restrictions and emailing the flight company but I'm not getting responses. I guess I understand because they're going through their own difficulties. It's not any clearer for them.

Let me just think about the worst-case scenario in terms of training. Okay the training is extended. Maybe I have to do an exam later on in the year? A couple of months later?

I'm trying to figure it out so I've got some certainty. That's the problem though, there is no certainty. There is no stability. This is an ever-evolving situation that we have to figure out as it comes. What do we fall back on when the entire structure of society is challenged? I mean for me I look to faith.

We look to history even to see what happened in previous circumstances. People keep talking about the influenza pandemic 100 years ago.

2nd April 2020

I'm trying to make the best of the little things right now. I may get some takeaway soon. Trying to work on my gym technique. It was payday recently which is always nice.

I don't know what's happening right now with our training or even our exam. Our training may be extended; I don't really like that.

I mean there are benefits to it too. I could be in a worse place. But right now, everything is up in the air. We don't know what's going to happen in the future.

Interesting event recently:
One colleague got a bit agitated with how our work patterns were being re-structured. Another more senior trainee stepped in and said *"think of our hospital colleagues – they're dying on the front line"*

The number of confirmed cases of COVID-19 has passed 1 million. That's quite a bad feat. I don't think this has fully impacted Britain; it's probably about to.

4th April 2020

I had some time off recently. I really needed to recuperate.

This extra day we have to work a week has been tough. We're coming in and working an extra day. Just the mental drain and uncertainty is a challenge.

We don't have any clarity on our future and we're having to work extra hard. We're not being paid extra for this. I do appreciate that we are in the business of caregiving. But we still have mortgages and bills to pay. I think a lot is up in the air right now; particularly for us. Everyone is trying to do their best.

I'm trying to work through my own weaknesses and feelings.

4th April 2020

It's rare that I do two entries on a day but I guess I needed to. It's therapeutic for me.

I'm thinking about what to do after this whole pandemic thing is over. Will I take a break? Go straight into work?

9th April 2020

It's Easter holidays and coronavirus is rampant. I guess it's brought all of the family closer together. Mum has been shielding during this time – she had cancer about 10 years ago; it was a very difficult time for us. We have to be extra careful for her. So I'm coming in, changing clothes, showering, and using a different entrance. I'm trying to stay a little away from her at times too. I haven't hugged her in a long time. I miss that.

My team has been very supportive at work. Really accommodating. I'm trying to figure out a routine. I'm going into work in different clothes too. Even my dad took some time off work for a little bit. I keep having to tell him that he needs to change his work routine too and he can't just meet lots of people.

I can see how this period will make a lot of difficulties for many families.

China ended the lockdown in Wuhan where it all began; that happened yesterday. They were allowed to leave for the first time in many days. We don't really have much information about what happened there. The pictures looked quite horrifying. Furthermore, when we see images of Italy it's very worrying how they're coping.

There are worse places to be in life right now than where we are, I guess.

11th April 2020

I'm trying to live in the present; if we live in the future or the past then we focus on something that doesn't exist. Obviously, I've got a lot of tension right now. I guess all I can really do now is watch and wait
.

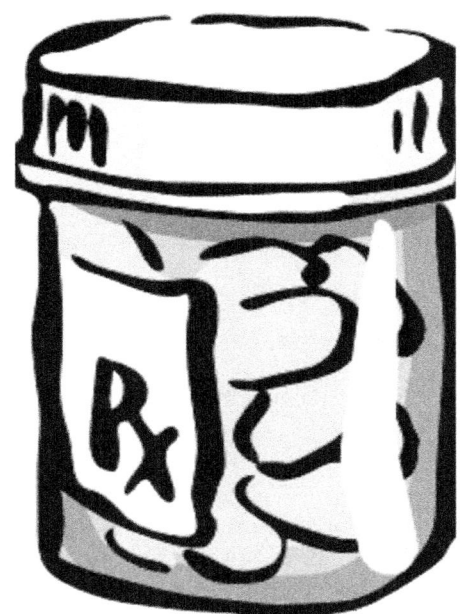

I believe yesterday the death toll exceeded 100,000 globally. That's a tenfold increase from March; it's only been a month. This does not seem to bode well.

13th April 2020

What I've started to do is to chronicle the things I'm looking forward to just to keep myself going.

We are really in the eye of the storm, right now. I feel it. That being said I'm enjoying my days off and I'm becoming accustomed to a new routine.

This is the new normal.

I'm trying to work out at home. I need to improve my skipping. I'm enjoying the TV shows that I watch. I'm just trying to find the little things that keep me going within this time. Obviously, there's a lot on my mind. I'm just trying to distract myself through this.

I've got some tension. I don't know what will come of this exam. I don't know what's going to happen with the marriage. I paid for the honeymoon. Will that go through?

On the other side I'm enjoying some of the television shows I'm watching. I'm looking forward to some things I've ordered. I've got the weekend coming up so that will be nice.

16th April 2020

If I'm honest there's not much new today.

The current lockdown has been extended. Another couple of weeks; at least.

We don't know what's going to happen; we're already thinking about a second wave and will that occur in the winter? What would that look like? Will that happen? Do we need another lockdown?

I'm happy with some of the things I've ordered which is good. I like the belt that I bought too. I'm just trying to find something to look forward to in all of this.

I've got to keep on keeping on.

By yesterday there were more than 2 million cases worldwide of coronavirus. It's impacting everything; I think even the 2020 Tour de France was cancelled. Everything is becoming affected. I'm sure it will affect the average person too in unforeseen ways.

18th April 2020

If I'm honest, right now I've got to be prepared that they're going to extend training for another 1 to 2 months, at least. Maybe more.

We haven't got a plan yet for all the wedding events – everything is still up in the air.

I'm trying to make the best of a bad situation. Obviously, I can't go to the gym so I've learnt to put up with doing some work on my skipping.

It's scary looking at what's happening. It's picking up pace rapidly. I think we're past 100,000 Covid related deaths just yesterday. It's not hit us so hard yet but it looks like it's going to?

Life is becoming a little bit monotonous. I'm trying to be as calm as I can. In some ways this really hasn't been that much of a change for me; obviously I can't socialise and I'm going to work as I normally would do. Spending my time mostly in the same ways. I think I've been okay with not socialising so far. It's probably brought us together as a family.

I think the overall headline for me here is that I may have to wait until December 2020 for this year of work to finish and to qualify as a GP.

It's the holy month of Ramadan soon. This is a month for spiritual enhancement more than anything.

Normally I learn a few more passages of the Holy Quran. I try to eat cleaner too. I try to purify myself internally. I believe that's exactly what this month is about. Reprioritising.

In this month we wake up early, pray early and then do not eat/drink until the evening/sundown. I often find this does my voice in as it's dry and as a GP we speak all day. It has been a little bit disconcerting to be honest.

Not eating doesn't really bother me. It's more about having the energy lag. I think it's the lack of coffee that does me in. I remember when I worked in a mental health hospital one of the nurses commented that you look like you lost your mojo when you fast. That was during **Ramadan!**

19th April 2020

Today I've been doing some mental calculations as to where some of my costs have been going. I'm thinking about maybe buying some new clothes. The little things we have to look forward to eh? There are some small victories and joys.

I think the in-laws are coming round to the idea that things are going to change with the wedding dates. We might do a little function at our house instead.

21st April 2020

I'm weighing up this whole job. Being a doctor. It's nice to have regular pay and a friendly environment. The team is very supportive. At the same time there are limits to my freedom. It's a regular commitment you have to have. It's all particularly tough now. I enjoy the intellectual and people side of it though.

This whole virus thing is so new – it's such a shock to the system. Mum is shielding for the next three months. I'm trying to be very rigorous about hand hygiene. But it's always going to be a worry, isn't it? I think we're all worried about bringing an infection back home.

At the same time I'm really enjoying out of hours medical work and Emergency Medicine. Maybe I can look into this further in the future.

I had a tough encounter at work today. I emphasised the importance of being calm to myself. Frankly that got me through the day. Ultimately, it's more effective and now I am calmer. I know I'll sleep better. I can only put all of this to God. It just reinforces the importance of being calm and dealing with the situation in the right manner.

I really now understand the importance of how we speak – I mean controlling our words. I've picked up the PlayStation again. I'm working hard on my diet too.

I'm spending more time with nature which makes me think. I love nature. I wish I spent less time on screens. It's given me an understanding about myself and what I'd like to do for the rest of my life. This internal reflection has been good for me spiritually. Even whilst training physically at home I've been working on new exercises and trying to gain strength.

22nd April 2020

I've got a couple of sources of tension today. I'm not sure what's going on with the wedding. Again, not sure what's happening with the exam or our career progression.

I feel constrained. If I'm honest I haven't felt like this in a really long time. So much is up in the air. How do you balance yourself when everything is uncertain?

Trying to stay positive, I'm looking forward to getting paid soon. I've got my eye on a couple of things. I am looking forward to when things eventually come through with Pernia. I'm enjoying my hobbies.

One thing I have realised about all of this is that shouting doesn't work. It never seems to work. If I deal with things Islamically then things do get a bit better. I feel more in control; by which I mean morally. I don't want to say something I regret.

At the same time, I've got so much going for me. I'm looking around at this coronavirus crisis. I've got a nice job. I'm almost finished with my training, regardless, whenever it may be. I'm so glad that I found Pernia. To some degree I'm carrying on as normal; I can't say that for everyone else with what's going on. I'm happy I got some money back on my tax return - that's always welcome!

If I'm honest I've got a little bit bored today and I was looking up some old colleagues of mine online. I was very troubled by what I saw and it made me aghast. One of the junior doctors who I worked with was going on to be a very promising doctor. He was an incredibly hard worker; he was very committed. He was always very pleasant. Very sweet, gentle, but a hard-working man. He was now in a care home at such a young age. No words to express how tragic the situation is or how I feel. It makes me feel so grateful for what I have.

I'm not so good at dealing with stress. All of the stuff piles up. Sometimes I find it hard to cope and make sense of all of it. Then comes my reaction and it's not always the best reaction.

We don't give enough thanks for what we do have. Wonder why that is?

23rd April 2020

I'm just expecting that I won't have my exam any time soon. It's just a bit of a stress because I clearly revised for it. I just wanted to get out of the door and work as a GP.

I must fix this in my mind!

25th April 2020

In this holy month of Ramadan I'm trying to read a bit more. I am trying to learn more of the Holy Quran. This was the month when the Holy Quran was first revealed so it has a very special significance for us. Each day obviously I look forward to eating and stopping the fast. That's a highlight!

There are so many benefits to fasting; it is like a reset or a detox each year that happens. It's definitely something I want to try and take forward. I've definitely been praying a lot harder in coronavirus. Haven't we all?

I must be prepared to extend my training. Ultimately when things fall out of our hands, we must put our faith in something else. For me that's where Islam comes in.

I'm looking forward to seeing Pernia soon.

On the other side of things, the global death toll from Covid has passed 200,000. It doesn't seem so long ago this was just a small mess. This is rapidly becoming a major issue across the world.

26th April 2020

In **Ramadan** usually I have learnt to cook better; although my family is still sceptical about my culinary skills. I really enjoyed cooking with my housemates at medical school. Those were fun times. My friends were solid cooks so I learnt a lot! Maybe one day I would like to do a proper cooking course.

I've got a long list of things I need to do.

Stop procrastinating!

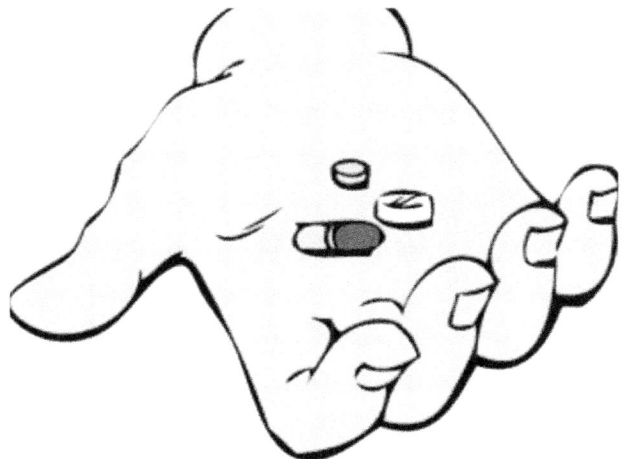

29th April 2020

I feel I made the best out of the circumstances. I'm thinking of all the other things I should be grateful for.

This holy month has definitely brought us together as a family as well. I do feel a bit more spiritually intact. In fact, I think this whole pandemic has done this. We've all made a concerted effort to spend more time together.

I'm waiting back on the refund for the honeymoon. I was really looking forward to going to Santorini. Hey ho! Will need to do something else.

29th April 2020

Right now, I'm going through a period of uncertainty in relation to my job. I mean at the same time at least I have one. I'll be so glad to have Pernia. I'm just thinking about this exam too. It will clearly happen at some point. My thoughts are just everywhere at the minute.

I really do feel some resentment building up. It's not helpful. At least I've identified it and can do some work to remove it. It is certainly not beneficial for me being pulled in all these different directions.

I think just the nature of the situation is worrying me. Resentment goes up and down; it's not anyone's fault but obviously I feel aggrieved about the whole thing. About everything.

I mean it's a lot worse for other people. I'm complaining about working too much but I know people have lost their jobs and would love to work the number of days that I do. Sometimes I think I live in my head too much. I always try and overthink; one of my supervisors said something like that to me once. You can't plan everything out. Life is 90% what happens to you and 10% how you react.

I do look forward to having some time off coming up. At the same time maybe the month of May could be a little harder. I really feel journaling has helped. It helps to get things out. Sometimes I just don't feel it beneficial to complain to people.

30th April 2020

I keep getting caught up in the moment. Sometimes I think when I dwell on my feelings that leads to resentment. Mostly about what's going to happen with the exam and going forward with progression.

I conclude it's best to be easy-going. Easier said than done though.

Has me questioning my career choices....

I'm looking forward to payday. I'm really getting back into PlayStation which has been great; I need my hobbies just to get through this. Some light leisure.

30th April 2020

I'm reflecting back on Ramadan and what I have gained out of it so far. I do feel I became a little bit more flexible mentally about the fact that I may not become a GP this year and the wedding may be postponed. I definitely feel a lot less resentment.

I'm finding writing all this down helpful.

I'm just thinking, in the long term what difference does it make? I'll be able to have my freedom and work as I wish soon.

I'm thinking about what I would like to do in the future. Maybe work a couple of days a week and focus on my other hobbies in the rest of the week; have a couple of days off, travel and such forth. Money has never really been my driving factor. I'm very fortunate to have a job with constant income. I think it's really about contentment for me and just being settled. I think the millennial generation really exemplifies this.

1st May 2020

I definitely feel a lot less resentment and a lot more flexibility. That's taken some work and some time. Sometimes I think we just live in our own head too much. We look at everything from every angle. I certainly do – sometimes that's not helpful.

All of our challenges can be overcome by our attitude. If we can change our attitude then we can change our environment. I think the thing most on my mind is about the fact that lockdown and the current coronavirus pandemic has interrupted our higher training and career progression.

I think it's interesting in some ways. Primarily it's not the money that's the issue here. It's sort of everything around the job. I'm curious to identify the problem but I don't know how to fix it.

I was just trying to think of mental devices to deal with it all. Okay I have all these challenges about the current work situation, exam situation and the wedding being held off (or the honeymoon!) but how does one cope?

But maybe I could put down my resentment backpack and put on my flexible spectacles. Maybe there's a good way of looking at all of this. It's just dead weight that's not helping me and I'm carrying it around. It's slowing me down. I need to look at this anew.

Maybe there is another way to look at this; in a way that I need to see properly. **I like that – flexible spectacles!**

2nd May 2020

Today I really don't feel I have the energy. It's one of the few, rare days I feel like this.

The positives are really good though I guess right now. I bought some stuff online. I've got a tax refund. Eid is coming soon. I'm enjoying some of my hobbies. Little victories.

5th May 2020

Don't live in your head! I think that's the other extreme of all of this. I really appreciate the outlet I have in writing a journal though.

We are looking at pictures and videos of Italy. It seems the intensive care units have been hit incredibly hard. It's quite worrying for us to look at that because some of the talk is that we're only a few weeks behind them. How will we cope?

The death toll in the United Kingdom has become high. It's been upwards of 30,000 people. These are just numbers, but these were ultimately people's lives and families that were affected.

It's not even just the old people that are affected; we are seeing pictures and videos on social media of young people saying *"don't take this virus lightly"*.

6th May 2020

Something happened today that made me realise I don't take criticism so well. I think part of this is the bigger picture for me. I need to be a bit more flexible. That resentment sometimes just drags me down.

I think what is unsettling is the job uncertainty – as a potential I could have up to 3 weeks left on my job or up to 6 months. I don't know.

That voice in your head sometimes can be unsettling. We all have to work against that; it's better to get it onside than go to war with it.

7th May 2020

I've turned to retail therapy a little bit to get through this lockdown. I was doing my calculations and accounting as to what I need to set aside for the future.

It's been helpful having little things to look forward to.

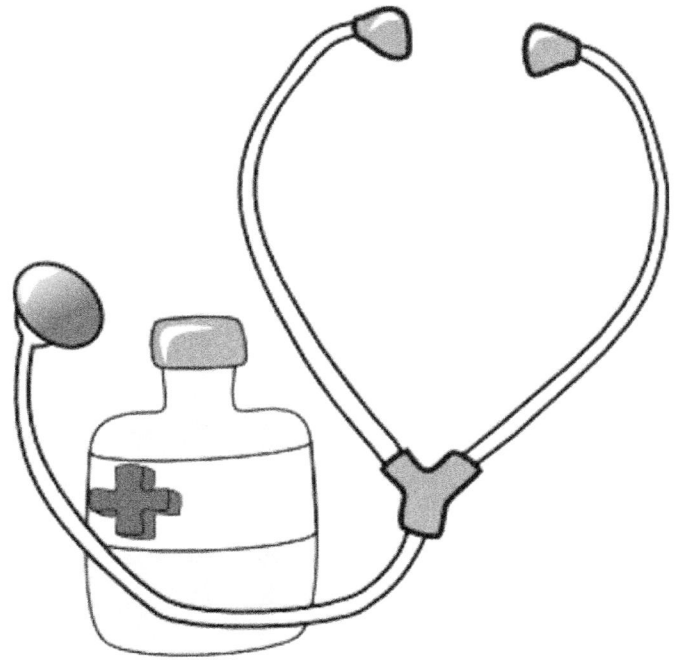

8th May 2020

Today I feel really contented. I asked myself *"why wouldn't I?"* Some of the formal marriage procedures are done. Technically I'm legally married. We had our registration but the other functions were postponed. I feel blessed even if the major functions are delayed past the summer.

I'm waiting to get my money back on my honeymoon. I know Pernia is very upset about not having all of the functions in the way that she wanted.

The fact that some things have now gone my way, it makes me feel really bad about complaining before. It makes me feel ashamed if I'm honest. It's given me a little bit more clarity. Ultimately, I want to try and act calmly when the situation is wanting.

8th May 2020

I think over time my anger has decreased. I don't know if resentment is common. Maybe resentment is the wrong word or maybe it's too strong a word; I'm deeply embedded in my feelings about this whole thing and so many things.

I'm happy too though. In a couple of days, it's going to be the end of the holy month of Ramadan and I'll get to see my wife.

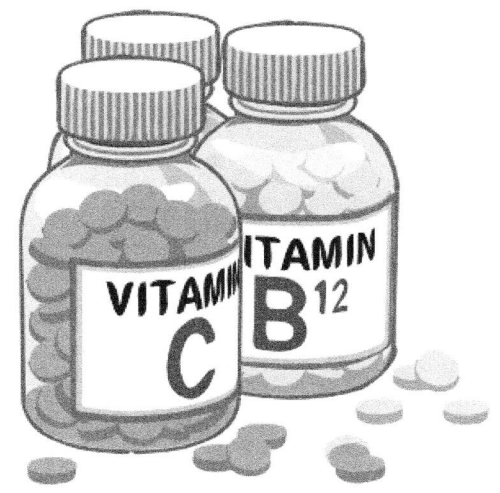

9th May 2020

Today I feel like I almost have no worries. How strange some of those same things are there that are not settled but I feel better. It's all about mentality. I'm glad for what I have.

This whole thing is a rollercoaster of emotions.

I think I just want to be prepared for whatever happens in any way that it does.

14th May 2020

The last 10 days been tough – obviously with all the things that are still going on. There is no clear outcome to many things.

I have the next few days off which gives me a bit of stability. This time off is crucial and much needed. We don't give ourselves enough of a break. We do not do enough self-care.

The government made all these announcements that PPE is coming. We haven't really seen that on the front line. Our wonderful patients have donated PPE. This is a nationwide phenomenon from what I gather.

15th May 2020

We now have a new exam format called the Remote Consultation Assessment. I'm glad something is on the way; it sounds like it's been very difficult for the Royal College of GPs to put this together but I'm glad that they did. I'm sure I can get it together and be out of the door by August to become a GP. At least it's a way out. I'll get another chance. Fulfilling a dream.

It does make me think about trying to make this positive. I'm usually stuck in my feelings for about a day. Often, I find that I'm better a day or so later.

I'm trying to save up to buy a property. It seems quite unrealistic to save up £60-£70,000; I don't know how long that will take. Maybe in the future I could do that but I think just right now I can't do that. Maybe I have to reassess in a bit. I just wonder how people do it in this society – it's not easy. It seems like society is not built to help those looking to get on the property ladder.

15th May 2020

I feel very fortunate that my wife has got a job nearby us. We may end up working together. So many times when doctors marry one another, one partner can be placed far away. That means we can live together and that's really important for the first year of our marriage. That means I can also look after her.

It can be quite disconcerting moving to a new area and starting a high pressure job like being a doctor particularly at a young age. I don't really appreciate all of this enough to be honest. It was so long ago for me but when I think back about those times. I recall the difficulties of it.

Okay, I appreciate the wedding won't go ahead as planned but something is better than nothing. As long as something can happen?

I'm just very grateful that there is a way for the exam to be sorted and for me to hopefully pass that.

It will be really nice that it will be the Eid festival soon. It's usually a time we get together and that will be lovely especially with what's happening right now.

Still waiting on the airline to get back to me on the refund.

16th May 2020

I've got a little bit of tension about this new exam now. It's going to take a lot of time. It's good that there are controlled submissions and that we have loose guidelines. But it's going to be a tough couple of weeks ahead.

I'm really going to have to knuckle down.

I've always thought whenever you lose, don't lose the lesson. Although there have been a number of challenges during this time, I've just tried to make the most of it.

I break my life down into different domains. Then I want to work on each of them. That means to improve my spiritual, physical, financial and career prospects.

18th May 2020

As predicted this exam is proving a little bit tricky. I need to get 13 recorded cases in a space of a few very short weeks. I think it's great that we have a possibility to try and get through to become GPs by August. it will be tough to get all of this done.

Ramadan is the month of patience. I really tried to take that in. I always believe that the right things happen, but are we in the right state? Where exactly am I meant to be? How do we embrace what comes?

19th May 2020

There's a lot going on right now in terms of coronavirus. One patient I knew died: I wasn't too sure exactly what was happening with that patient. That hit me hard. I discussed this case endlessly to see if there were any learning points for me – most definitely there always are. I always want to improve. I'm glad that person passed away peacefully.

I'm really looking forward to the holy festival of Eid and the end of fasting. Hopefully payday should be soon. I look forward to spending some time with Pernia.

We're not living together, so I only get to see her at her house. She's now in her final year just finishing up her medical studies. She will be a doctor soon too if she finishes her exams. She felt unwell recently; she may have had the virus. I felt very helpless hearing how she was and she was miles away from her. I'm just glad she recovered.

I'm just reflecting on what happened with this recent death. This made me re-think about when things are unclear. Once a palliative care consultant said to me *"we don't know how to process death"* as a species. That was a very interesting discussion.

I think recently the global death toll passed 300,000 people. That's really worrying.

19th May 2020

If we fail to get the relevant cases what happens? It's a whole new thing. Will the training year be extended? We can try it again in December? I don't know.

Ultimately, at the end of day it's not the end of the world if I don't get through this exam. I just want to get through at some point, specialise and become a GP.

I know people are seriously struggling. I'm so glad to have worked. There are people that have lost jobs during this pandemic. I think it's important to step back. For me personally to pray on it is important. These are not untenable circumstances.

Yes, it's uncomfortable but I can definitely get through this.

20th May 2020

I feel a little bit calmer around this exam now I'm a little bit into it.

Patience…

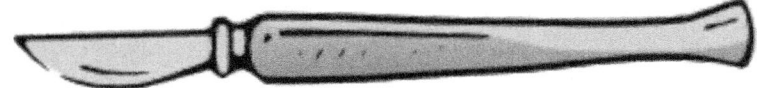

21st May 2020

This has been a difficult month. Looking for a way out.

I feel a bit calmer about the exam. One thing that is good is that I can leave it all at work. I'll just record everything. It's really good I've got the groundwork done. I've done my best for now.

I'm really trying to work on my character. If I don't react to any of these challenges positively then they're just wasted chances. I've lost the opportunity that way. One thing I've seen is that when I shout, it never seems to work with anyone.

I need to stay calm. It doesn't do me any good and it really disturbs my mental state. It disturbs my equilibrium. I need to control myself and I will always be happier after.

Can I honestly say I would do anything different? I don't think I would change any of my circumstances. I did my best in every single moment. I guess that gives me some reassurance.

24th May 2020

Patience always wins.

My mum was quite for it. She would come out and clap. I thought it was wonderful she showed this kind of community spirit. It's bringing us together. In our neighbourhood we have never really done this kind of thing.

24th May 2020

Figuring out this exam is a little bit difficult. I think I've got the trial period out of the way. Now I'm just trying to record and get as many cases as I can. The thing is to get it within a short time period.

I love Eid. It celebrates the end of the month of Ramadan where we fast. It's rooted in the story of Abraham and his sacrifice. We get the family together and have food. I listened to a sermon which related his story. We progress in life by putting a knife to our desires and sacrificing them. Sacrificing our desires means spiritual progress.

It's been nice and enjoyable to be able to eat again normally.

My anxiety levels about this exam are a bit down.

25th May 2020

It's now after Ramadan and I'm just trying to adjust to that life. I'm definitely little bit less anxious.

I'm working on trying to have the best routine I can. Trying to maximise on everything. It's almost like Ramadan was a reset for me. I definitely took away some good habits so that's really good to know too.

I've tried to adjust my diet a little bit so I have an early dinner then I'm trying to add to my cardio.

What we are seeing from America is horrendous; I can't believe this video I saw of this poor man with a police officer's knee on his neck. He even called out for his mother. That's how desperate he was. How can things like this happen?

I seem to have more questions than answers at the minute.

28th May 2020

I feel the last couple of days I've had the same old concerns. Same stuff about the exam and trying to record for it. I look forward to the marriage. I think hopefully we can have some kind of function later on in the year.

I'm just going from payday to payday trying to make something here.

I've been looking back at the past couple of days; there have been so many protests and riots. There's been so much violence and police brutality in America. I think we look to America for so many things but we have to say this is wrong. I'm just so surprised something like this can happen.

30th May 2020

I have noticed the days that I don't journal, I don't feel so well. Those are the days that I need to do it on to be honest. I mean ideally every day.

I thought having a day off yesterday was relaxing. Much needed. I think we don't do enough self-care in the society. I think that is the case especially for health workers.

I'm thinking of similar key workers who work such long hours, have to pay a mortgage/rent and look after their families. Then on top of that one has to try to look after one's mental health. To do that self-care and to take care of oneself is physically not so easy.

What I'm saying is that those key workers are the ones getting ill; interestingly it's not so easy for them to take time off. They have to work. If we look at those key workers in the shops, buses, and hospitals it is mostly immigrants doing these jobs for lower pay. We don't all have the luxury of isolating.

I'm getting somewhere with my recordings and preparing for the exam. I was just thinking about all the blessings that I have which include my family, some savings and having a mental framework to deal with the challenges that I face.

1st June 2020

Surely there is ease after hardship
Aye, surely there is ease after hardship

The Holy Quran
Chapter 94: When the Hearts Become Open

After hardship there is ease; that's a verse of the holy Quran. I think it's very profound. Even when I went for my daily walk around the practice today, I thought the exact same thing. Someone had put a painting which had sunshine coming out the clouds. It'll be okay in the end.

I think it makes writing something down all the more important because I have to remember the good days too. It's okay sometimes to not be okay.

I'm trying to move positively. That takes effort though at times and other times it's easier.

2nd June 2020

I'm making slow progress with the exam. Maybe I have about 5 cases out of the 13 that I need. In terms of work, I mean it's relatively much the same.

My trainer has been very kind and informed the whole practice that my mother is shielding because of her previous background therefore I will not be seeing patients. I was asked to see a patient by a nurse; she didn't know that my mother was shielding therefore I saw them. I then told her afterwards. I was very nervous about this. We're all so worried about our families, understandably so.

However, this whole thing is evolving. I'm not sure when I will be able to work normally. I don't want to make it a difficult thing for anyone else and ask them to do my work.

I'm still waiting on my airline to give me some compensation back.

It's been enjoyable having some time off. I look forward to seeing Pernia next weekend. I've really been counting down the days to this.

3rd June 2020

I'm sitting back analysing this exam. To get 13 cases for submission looks like quite possible. I'm glad that I have a date. I'm glad I have something in the end of sight. I just have to keep up my progress now. I'm having to come in on top of my extra days for other extra days just to get the recordings in.

I never want to look back and think what if?

I just feel I'm waiting on a lot of still. I'm waiting on what will happen with this exam and trying to get money back from the airlines for the honeymoon.

I'm still a little bit anxious to be honest. I'm trying to use this time to recalibrate. At the same time, I know things will get done. They always get done.

I've got a lot to look forward to. I do look forward to spending time with Pernia. I'm trying to work hard in the meantime. Furthermore, I'm quite glad I made some recent changes; I'm reading a bit more. I've made some dietary changes and I'm a bit more spiritually elevated.

Slow steps eh?

4th June 2020

I'm feeling excited about seeing Pernia. I'm feeling anxious though about my exam.

It's important to put in hard work. Be prepared.

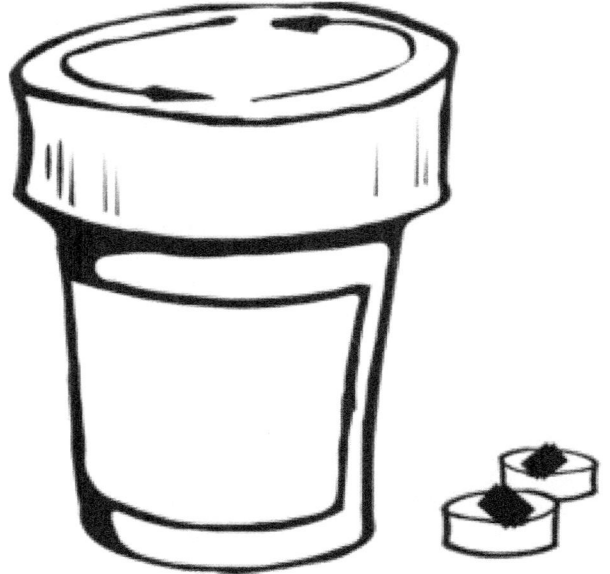

6th June 2020

I'm still a little bit tense because of this exam. Still trying to figure it out.

I think this is the first time I've documented that I'm actually a little anxious in lockdown. I'm looking forward to working in a normal job. Possibly looking forward to the future too. I mean I have been tensed at times. But actually, being cooped up has made me anxious. This is a new thing. Usually, I'm so on the go it's not a problem.

It's been a good time for me to reflect.

8th June 2020

We postponed the marriage functions; it's official. We've done the formal registration but there were meant to be a number of events that Asian families do. We have had to postpone them for now.

I'm not sure what's going to happen. It's not even clear if we'll be allowed to do them. Obviously, it's cost a lot of money. Obviously, Pernia was very excited, and now it looks like it won't happen. I mean of course so was I too. It shows me you can do all the planning in the world but sometimes things just go a totally different way.

It will be really nice that Pernia will come home with me next week nonetheless anyways. I've got some time off too; it was meant to be a honeymoon but I do really look forward to spending time with her.

The number of confirmed Covid cases seems to have passed 7 million. That's incredible and not in a good way.

10th June 2020

I'm very, very grateful to have met Pernia. I'm very grateful to have all the things that I have. Too many favours to count. I really truly believe in prayer and my prayers have been answered.

These things always make me feel that I need to be more patient. I feel ashamed because I didn't have enough patience.

I need to keep going. I need to try to strengthen myself.

17th June 2020

Mum had some symptoms: just a sore throat kind of thing and a runny nose. I was really worried about her. With her background of cancer that's the worrying bit. She is shielding. I really want to make sure she's okay. Thankfully her test came back negative though which is really, really great. That was a real scare.

We really haven't played loose with any of the rules. We try to be as strict as we can in terms of adhering to the guidelines.

Despite all of this going on I'm just very grateful for everything. I see a lot of my other friends and colleagues are having an incredibly difficult time.

I see the end in sight at least for this exam. Some of my other projects are going well too.

I've tried to change my diet during this time. I just felt we're going through this trial and I wanted to make the most of it.

Always turn your losses into victories.

17th June 2020

It's rare for me to make two entries in the same day but hey ho I thought I should do it. I feel really happy. I tried to make the best out of everything that I can. The Arabic word for patience (صَبْر) entails more than just simply patience but also perseverance. It's quite a holistic meaning.

Pernia has got her job allocation in the local hospital. It's where I work as well. That's really a blessing. She could've been posted anywhere. I'm really grateful for that. Obviously, that's a big transition for her to leave her family and to come start working as a junior doctor. I really hope I can guide her in that.

I got given the money back from my honeymoon. Payday is coming soon too. Little victories.

18th June 2020

I've really enjoyed this week that's far. Things seem to finally be going right, despite everything else around us not working out so well.

At the present I'm just trying to stay focussed. Whenever things get tough, I think KIM:
Keep
It
Moving

I've started thinking about touching up our little flat a little bit more. When Pernia comes it can be ready for her.

I was thinking about the tribulations that I have had – this included about mum's health scare, the honeymoon money, the exam and the wedding being pushed back. Eventually these all did sort themselves out, albeit in different ways. Unexpected ways.

The one thing that I keep coming back to is to have patience. That is the tool. But it just takes a long time to absorb that and understand that.

It will be okay in the end. But that's in the end.

20th June 2020

I feel a little bit stressed about this exam. Some of my submissions are not suitable and my trainer is away. I've still got to get some recordings. Deadline is coming up soon.

Right now, it comes down to faith. So much of this thing is out of my hands. Look at what's going on around the world; it's all out of our hands. I can only do my best – I'm just worried my best isn't good enough.

21st June 2020

I feel very blessed. It's interesting how things change so much in a day. I feel I'm on the way to getting my exam sorted. Hopefully I'll be finished with my training soon and I'll be a fully qualified GP. I'm looking forward to payday. I feel incredibly grateful for my health and that I've been safe thus far.

You know, there are so many things that I feel thankful for. A place to stay, some savings, my job, my faith and my wife. I wish I was more grateful and I was more patient.

I just feel that no matter what happens there is always benefit. We do not always see it clearly in the heat of battle. The only time I ever seem to win is when I show patience.

23rd June 2020

I feel tension sometimes can be a never-ending cycle. It begins in an awkward way which then compounds and then exacerbates underlying issues. So, it's important to try get out of that before it gets worse.

I think way too much. Over-think I mean. One of my friends in America once said that when you live inside your head it's really tough. It's true. It doesn't help me. Why is it that we focus more on negative energy than anything else? I do find mindfulness beneficial, although I never really practised it too much – our thoughts run wild and we must control them. That is the same for many other things.

I think I finally got all my recordings together for this new exam. We submit 13 cases and that's our sign off to become fully-fledged GPs. Now it's just about having faith.

Stay calm I tell myself. I get so worked up; I need to talk myself down more. Often, I can work myself up a lot and that's the problem.

24th June 2020

I'm looking forward to this exam being over. I've got some days off coming up and payday too. When I've got those positive things to look forward to it helps me dampen down my ruminations. I hear this a lot from patients: ruminations are worse and they can't sleep; definitely the same for me too. Then my mind gets going about the negative things and I can't process them.

I believe nothing is really ever as bad as it feels in your head. The anticipation is always worse than anything.

I think mental health as a concept is more prominent now than before; probably because we are locked up with ourselves.

I was reflecting recently: many of my friends are going through relationship problems in some way or another. I feel very blessed to have my wife.

I'll look at some of my closest friends who lost their mothers to cancer whilst mine survived. I strongly firmly believe it was so many prayers that saved her. I appreciate that sounds wild, being a doctor myself. That's my belief. So many studies have actually shown the efficacy of prayer. I believe it's not that far off then.

24th June 2020

I have to finalise my submissions for the new exam. I've been in two extra days just to make sure my submission list looks great. One day I was hoping to see extra patients and another day I was uploading all my submissions and then the power cut off; almost everything that could go wrong did go wrong!

Things are slowly coming together.

We make so many plans and it's often the smallest of things that can throw them out of sync. Our plans don't take into account how many factors can go wrong.

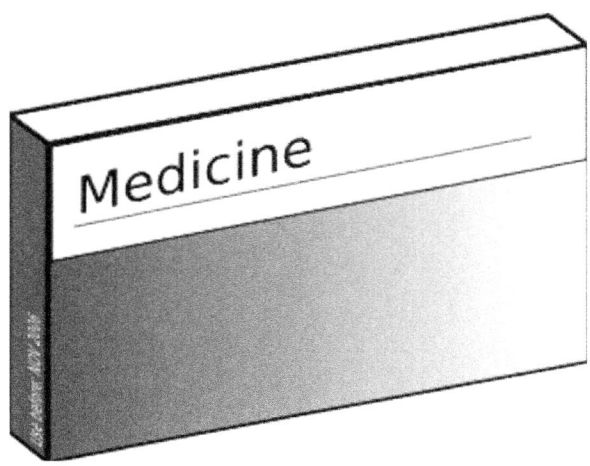

26th June 2020

Obviously, this period has been very difficult for everyone so I've tried to turn internally. I want to use every opportunity to better myself because otherwise it's just time wasted. I tried to use this time to improve my diet, commit to skipping, and improve my spirituality. I'm glad I've definitely come out of this a lot stronger in every way.

Even as religious people we often just seek to get things from God but we don't really focus on actually building a relationship. Ultimately the priority is to actually build that relationship. Just strengthening ourselves mentally and freeing ourselves from our desires is tough.

I appreciate not everyone will have the same sense of religion but I'm sure everyone believes in something in some way – whether that's our consciousness, fate or some sense of spirituality. That is something we can all improve on.

1st July 2020

I'm very happy.

I haven't written anything recently because I've been busy. That's often a tendency of mine. Only when I start feeling the pressure do I feel the need to commit to writing anything down. I really recommend journaling to every patient who I speak to because I find it so beneficial.

I'm thinking about the future. The end is in sight. What happens when I'm no longer a GP trainee and a GP? How will I work? I have some projects I would like to focus on.

Reflecting back now; all that hard work has paid off.

Lockdown is easing – life is returning to a mild normality. Now I think I did not see all the positives before.

It's just incredible how our mind limits itself and is not open to change. Time is the changer.

4th July 2020

It's been like a dream recently. I got the money back from my honeymoon. I've got my submissions in for the exam. I've got some days off. I feel so grateful that Pernia's job is nearby. My mum has been safe during this time. I've got an income coming in.

The one thing all of this has taught me is the value of prayer, patience and perseverance.

6th July 2020

Today I made a mental list of all the things I'm very grateful for. It was a very long list. Needless to say, whenever I go through this it really does make me feel better.

7th July 2020

Waiting.

Patiently waiting for my results to see if I can become a GP.

9th July 2020

I know I did my best. I put my best foot forward. I have my faith. I know my trainer did her best too. I'll keep on waiting. I need to think positively though.

Reflecting back on my entries it seems like I was going through the same emotions when I sat my first exam way back at the start of the year. I am just waiting for the results like I was before.

12th July 2020

I got a little nervous today. After some time that did settle with reflection. Then I felt positive.

I remember when I worked in a mental health unit, they talked about undergoing certain mental techniques to try and break the rhythm of negative thoughts. Easier said than done. Afterwards though I did feel more positive when I thought through that.

Ultimately there is goodness and wisdom in everything but it depends upon how we react to things. I really believe I could not have done anything differently.

13th July 2020

This exam is really taking up my mental faculties. I've done everything I can.

I think about my friends and colleagues who have failed; some of them failed three or four times. I strongly believe they were far cleverer than I am.

I think back to when I was applying for medical school. Our careers advisor told me not to apply because I was not predicted a full flush of 'A's'. I was not predicted an 'A' grade in Chemistry. Nonetheless I applied; one rejection came. I remember I was in Pakistan when that happened. I remember I was offered a biomedical degree and my mum said I could take that. Two more rejections came. It was my last chance, then I remember I got a call when I was watching a film in the basement back in England. I couldn't believe it. I couldn't take it seriously that a medical admissions panel was calling me for an interview. My dad handed me the phone.

Very much like an adolescent and a juvenile I said *"is this a joke?"*. I was so excited. I remember my interview well. Ultimately it was the best university for me. It was a wonderful time. I ended up getting that 'A' in chemistry against all odds. A 'B' in Biology though!

I know I did all I could. I tried to change my style as much as I could. I came in extra days. I did five or six times more recordings than I needed. I really cannot think of anything else I could have done.

14th July 2020

It's the day before my results. I kept a fast today.

I was thinking of how I wouldn't change very much about my life and how perfect things are; particularly how they all happened for the best. To me personally that's a sign of prayer.

I could not ask for a better life. In terms of my education, I had the best education that my parents worked hard to give me. Even at medical school I enjoyed myself. Throughout my GP training I was in my local hospital and I truly felt like I was serving my community.

When I had time out of training, I travelled the world and I studied abroad. I cannot think of a better job other than what I am doing.

I remember back when my mum was ill. She was in hospital for most of it. She was in and out of hospital afterwards with recurrent infections. Of course, we were really worried. That changed my life. That changed the way I think about things.

One of the seven deadly sins for the Romans was luxuria. It seems like I have so much and that came to mind. I just think of the things that I have; my mental health, my savings, my career, my physical health, living where I live and having the resources that I do.

14th July

I'll still keep working on my other projects including my book. I still have my freedom.

15th July 2020 AM
(pre-results)

It's the morning of results. I feel a bit calmer than yesterday. I kept a prayer and fasted yesterday.

Ultimately, I could only deal with what was in front of me. I went in extra days. I tried to change and take all the criticism on board to become a better doctor within a short time. I guess I feel confident and a little bit calmer.

I come back to that everything makes sense to me at this point. Now because of all of this I have a better knowledge and a better skill set.

Not everything comes easily. Sometimes things do but sometimes they don't…

15th July 2020 PM (pre-results)

Waiting on the results. It's billed as the last final exam we will ever have to do as doctors. Be prepared for anything; whether that's a pass now or four months more of work. I just need to get on with it. Ultimately a lot of this was out of my control.

I remember once I did an exam as an extra qualification. It came in two parts. I thought I had the essay in the bag; actually, I didn't. It was the practical exam that was straightforward. I failed that written assessment and then I had to re-do it again. Totally out of the blue.

15th July 2020
(post-results)

\+
Passed!!!!!!!!!

This is perfect. I could not see everything before; the wisdom behind it all. I'm very fortunate to have passed. Ultimately, I needed patience. This was a chance to increase that and improve myself as a person. I feel very blessed.

To celebrate I do have a list of things I would like to do: I would like to get my business off the ground. I'll start thinking about that.

I'm thinking about setting up a YouTube channel. I would like to get some websites off the ground for this exam now to help others too.
I would like to try and fast this Saturday.

I need to try and get to the gym regularly. I want to focus more on compound exercises. Working on my skipping. Maybe try a walk in the evening?

17th July 2020

I'm looking forward to going to Bath tomorrow with my friends. We were going to go to Bournemouth but that has been packed recently so we can't go there. No places to stay. It was meant to be an overnight lads thing. But my friends are pretty last minute.

There's been no social distancing. It seems that everyone has forgotten that they are in the middle of a worldwide emergency.

Now is the time for payback. To try and make myself better for those around me. To contribute in a positive way. I want to try and work harder on my other projects.

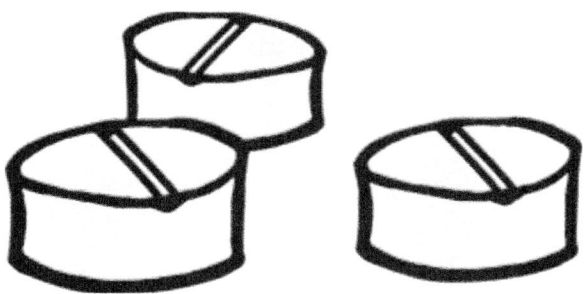

21st July 2020

Bath was so fun! It was so good to spend time with my friends in such a way! One of my circles of friends is so eclectic. Saeed is Saeed. Abdus Salam always has a tremendous sense of humour. I admire Hamza and his commitment and work ethos. HK is the guy everybody wants to be around. I never have a dull conversation with Rebs. Raza, Mirra, Obi, Mo and Arafat always make me smile. I always learn something when I'm with Kareem. Not to mention the countless others.

It's such a pretty place. We walked around a lot. The centre of the city and the outskirts are cute. We had a great time. Hope to do it again soon.

Now that I've passed my exam I'm thinking about the future. I need to get my indemnity sorted so I am insured to work as a GP. I want to try and make a logo for my company. I have to do a number of things to make sure I can actually work as a GP.

I'm thinking of putting together some resources for this exam. There's not a lot out there at the minute because it is so new.

I'm thinking about the future. It's a blessing in a way. I could work as a GP in hours, as a GP out of hours or even in Emergency Medicine.

25th July 2020

I haven't got any work as of yet for the next month. I'm trying to figure out how to get my parking permit for the local hospital too. I'm trying to go through the rigmarole of getting my company registered.

This is very much a transition phase. It will be over soon. There is so much going on. I'm trying to transition to a new job. Transition to married life. I want to work on other projects that I'm passionate about.

There is so much more on the way. There was certainly a little bit of uncertainty. That's how strength of character is tested though.

Smooth waters don't make a good sailor, as one of my seniors always says.

26th July 2020

Literally nothing I don't have.
I'm just grinding away on these projects
One step at a time…

31st July 2020

Lately I've been thinking about my savings and what to do. I think it's something a lot of young people are struggling with at the minute. Renting or buying? When renting it costs so much and a mortgage costs so much how is a young person meant to get on the property ladder?

I remember once one of my Master's classmates in London said *"I don't think I'll ever buy a property in London"*. This is when we were mature students at the age of 25-26. That was a surprise. He was a qualified teacher. What a shame.

It makes me think about how we view money; is there really a difference between a couple of thousand in the practical day-to-day terms? When it cannot always lend itself to be the basic foundation of a mortgage.

I think the way we view money is unhealthy. Maybe it's just me.

4th August 2020

My last day as a trainee GP. From tomorrow I will be a fully qualified GP!

I take life in a very stepwise measured approach. How can I improve? My diet, my gym routine my work etc…

Pernia will start work as well soon. I know she's been a little bit nervous. I was casting my mind back to when I was in her shoes. I am looking to see if I can manoeuvre my rota so I can work with her and ease her in. This way we can work together on the same day in the same hospital at the same time!

Poor thing, she's starting on night shifts too!

11th August 2020

I have got a lot of side projects and goals I want to commit to. I'm actually making them into a reality but it's proving so difficult; we have to just water our ideas each day until they grow. Like anything, I suppose?

I'm working hard on my three volumes of re-analysing Islam in America. I did a tour of America twice a few years ago: the locals, brothers and friends of mine were so supportive. They showed me around all the cities and gave me a place to stay. True brotherhood. I started reading about Islam in America and saw a lot of errors. There was a lot of room for improvement in terms of historical analysis. I wanted to put my Master's degree to use. Since 2018 I've been back and forth to America spending time researching, reading and studying. I've got about 500 pages written over 3 volumes. Thoroughly researched but I have a lot more reading to do.

I want to set up some service particularly to provide for mental health in many different languages. Something I struggled with myself. I remember when my grandfather and grandmother both had dementia. Both circumstances were very difficult to deal with because of the language barrier – trying to get carers to come to our home and look after them was tough. The burden on carers is unreal particularly when it is a relative.

Those were incredibly tough times; we had two goes of it. Firstly, my grandfather got severe dementia and then a few years later my grandmother did. That first time round I worked far away and was coming back on weekends to look after them. My mum was working full-time then too. She took part-time retirement when my grandmother started declining.

Those experiences will stay with me forever. I love the elderly. I wish I did more for them. It's so sad to see them put in homes and disregarded. Sometimes I think we forget that they can suffer with mental health issues too. I have seen in the elderly, it's a little bit different. It is not as always about having a low mood.

I miss my grandparents every single day. My grandmother was the sweetest lady. I really miss her especially.

15th August 2020

This is the last page of this little book I'm writing in – I mean the actual pages of this book. I wanted to compare it with the first page which was four months ago on the 15th April.

There were lots of sources of tension; that included failing the exam and the wedding. I wasn't sure about if I would get the money back from the holiday. However recently all of those have been resolved to some degree or another. I needed a space of four months. When you're going through the struggle, things just seem so tough.

Recently I read the worldwide number of Covid cases passed 20 million. This isn't going away. Is it going to get worse?

It seems like we are used to the coronavirus way of life now; that being said I think people are still getting used to social distancing. Whenever I drive through London the parks are always full; as are all the shops.

I wonder what the future holds…

Epilogue

After all was said and done everything was resolved. I eventually did pass my exam. I did become a GP. I did get married and Pernia did move in with me. We missed out on our honeymoon but we are together now.

I penned my diary just as a therapeutic release. Journaling really helped me get through the worst of times; as did my faith. They are both incredible tools. I advocate them for everyone. We are living in times when theoretically we should be more connected but sometimes, we feel further apart. Isn't that odd?

I Need A Second Opinion is the follow up to this diary. Things have changed dramatically since I wrote *Take A Deep Breath*. Now I'm working as a GP and an A&E doctor. Pernia has moved in; she's now working in her own right as a junior doctor. Follow the journey as we both chronicle our experiences during the second wave of the Covid-19 pandemic. This is an inside look at our relationship, workplace drama, mental health, stresses, highs and lows as doctors during the second wave of the Covid-19 pandemic.

Printed in Great Britain
by Amazon